Fleecy to Fit

All that you want to be
familiar with wellness
and fat misfortune

by 

Dr. Philip T. Steward

INTRODUCTION

In a world filled with an overwhelming barrage of information about fitness, wellness, and weight loss, ***"Fleecy to Fit"*** emerges as a guiding light in the often confusing and contradictory landscape of health and self-improvement. This book is not just another one-size-fits-all solution; it's a personal journey, a powerful narrative of transformation, and a comprehensive guide that will take you from a place of comfort and complacency to a state of vibrant health and well-being.

In the pages that follow, you will embark on an inspiring voyage of self-discovery, self-improvement, and self-empowerment. ***"Fleecy to Fit"*** is not about quick fixes or miracle cures. Instead, it's a testament to the remarkable capabilities of the human body and spirit, underlining that the path to wellness and weight loss is not about shedding pounds but gaining a new perspective on life.

The author, a dedicated wellness advocate, and experienced guide, shares his transformational journey from a place of 'fleecy' comfort to a state of being 'fit,' not just in body but in mind and spirit. Through their personal story and expertise, you will find the wisdom and motivation to initiate and sustain your unique journey toward a healthier, happier you.

This book is more than just advice on diet and exercise; it's an exploration of the psychology behind lifestyle changes, an illumination of the science underpinning wellness, and a revelation of the profound impact that self-care can have on your life. *"Fleecy to Fit"* will inspire you to take control of your health and redefine your relationship with your body, your habits, and your goals.

So, if you've ever yearned for a change if you've struggled to make sense of the countless wellness trends and fads, or if you simply desire a profound transformation in your life, *"Fleecy to Fit"* is your compass, guiding you on an exciting journey towards realizing your full potential. Get ready to shed the 'fleecy' layers that have held you back and embrace a future where 'fit' is not just a physical state but a holistic way of living. Your transformative journey starts here.

Table of Contents

Chapter 1

Grasping Wellbeing and Fat Misfortune

Wellbeing is the demonstration of pursuing sound routines consistently to achieve better physical and psychological well-being results so that rather than simply getting by, you're flourishing.

Regardless of whether you're not effectively battling with an emotional well-being issue, focusing on your emotional wellness is significant. Essentially, regardless of whether you haven't been officially determined to have an actual disease, it's as yet vital to focus on your body.

Well-being isn't the shortfall of stress or agony, however the predictable act of sound propensities to all the more likely further develop one's general prosperity. Well-being is a cognizant decision to flourish, rather than simply making a cursory effort in endurance mode.

Above all, health is a general condition of congruity in the body: psychological, physical, close to home, and profound.

All aspects of our being are interconnected. Our eating routine, practice, and other way of life propensities influence how our bodies feel. What our bodies feel means for our thought process. What we think means for how we act, and how we act directs the course of our lives.

Understanding and dealing with our general health is significant because everything in our bodies and lives is associated. At the point when one aspect drops askew, so can all the other things.

Fat misfortune, as the name implies, alludes to losing just an abundance of fat from the body. Fat, muscle, and water can play a part in weight reduction. Be that as it may, it can likewise happen because of different variables, for example, bone mineral or glycogen stores. Glycogen stores might be especially relevant for individuals following low-carb slims down.

Abundance muscle to fat ratio can adversely influence virtually every feature of life, including:
- diminished portability
- more unfortunately close to-home well-being and confidence
- expanded hazard of organ disappointment
- less fortunate circulatory wellbeing
- cxpanded hazard of coronary illness
- expanded chance of pressure cracks
- expanded hazard of strokes
- expanded hazard of tumors
- diminished sexual and regenerative wellbeing

Fat cells can go about as endocrine plants and produce chemicals that impact various cycles in the body — the majority of which lead to more fat amassing.

Past the strength, all things considered, conveying a lower muscle-to-fat ratio is in many cases considered more alluring and pleasing as the fundamental muscular structure is uncovered.

Further, conveying a lower muscle-to-fat ratio is favorable for the vast majority of sports contenders (notwithstanding sumo grapplers, linemen, and so on) as additional fat weight adds drag and extra opposition that should be survived.

Chapter 2

The most effective method to work out Marcos:

WHAT ARE MACROS?

Knowing how to utilize a full-scale mini-computer initially requires a comprehension of what macros are.

Set forth plainly, macronutrients are the majority of the matter that makes up the energy content of every piece of food you've at any point eaten. Protein, carbs(carbohydrates), and fat are the three 'macros' in your food, and they all add to your general calorie consumption in various ways.

Each macronutrient is estimated in grams and calories, which will add to your everyday objective. By tweaking the amount of each with a full-scale mini-computer, you can fuel your body for preparation - whether you're preparing for a photoshoot or a perseverance race.

In addition, figuring out how to count your macros implies you're giving close consideration to the make-up of your food. This assists you with becoming explicit about why you probably won't lose as much fat or acquiring as much muscle as you'd like.

Instructions on how to calculate Marcos

utilizing our full-scale mini-computer underneath can assist you with fitting your eating regimen to get granular on your benefits.

Protein: 4 Calories for each Gram
Named the 'muscle large scale', protein is comprised of long chains of amino acids. There are around 20 different amino acids generally tracked down in plant and creature proteins - in fluctuating extents, contingent upon the food - however just nine are 'fundamental', and that implies your body can't make them. Instances of high-protein food sources include fish, chicken, meat, Greek yogurt, tempeh, curds, eggs, jerky, lentils, and tofu.

Starches: 4 Calories for each Gram
Starches assume a critical part in your physical processes. They're the main energy hotspot for your body, which switches the large scale into glucose over completely to fuel your organs and muscles.
For this reason, perseverance competitors and exceptionally dynamic people follow a high-sugar diet. While both 'basic' and 'complex' carbs are sugars, there's a distinction between them.
Basic carbs are quick-processing sugars found normally in specific food varieties like white bread, products of the soil, yet additionally added to rolls, desserts, and cake. Complex carbs - likewise called

starches - contain longer chains of sugar atoms, which take more time to separate and give enduring energy. They're tracked down in peas, beans, entire grains, and veggies.

Fat: 9 Calories for every Gram

Fat gets negative criticism, however in truth, unsaturated fats - the structure blocks of fat, like omega-3 - are vital for your well-being. They assume a few significant parts, from safeguarding your organs to going about as synthetic couriers for proteins. Fat likewise assists your body with retaining nutrients A, D and E. Unsaturated fats, for example, olive oil, avocados, and nuts, assist with safeguarding your heart by controlling your cholesterol. You'll track down sound fats in slick fish, avocados, nuts, dairy items and creature fats.

Chapter 3

The most effective method to work out Calories

Calories are units of energy that a food or drink gives. You can ordinarily find carbohydrate levels recorded on food items, and wearables like the best fitness trackers permit you to screen the number of calories that you're consuming by doing various exercises. Certain food sources, like greasy, broiled, or handled food varieties, will quite often have more calories. Different food varieties, like new products of the soil, will generally have fewer calories. Nonetheless, a few sound products of the soil can be high in calories, while low-calorie food sources, like eating routine pop, offer no wholesome benefit.

Knowing the number of calories you need to consume every day might be useful for losing, acquiring, or keeping up with weight.

The BASAL METABOLIC RATE (BMR) is one of the strategies you can use in working out.

BMR is your pace of digestion (the change of calories and oxygen to energy) very still. It is the base degree of energy expected to support crucial capabilities like breathing, assimilation, and dissemination.

Verifying Your Everyday Calories
BASAL METABOLIC RATE (BMR) as a numeric worth. You are still up in the air by your sex, age, and body size, and working out this number educates you regarding the number of calories you consume simply being alive and alert.
The recipe for the BMR is very intricate.
Stage 1: Work out Your BMR
For ladies, BMR = 655.1 + (9.563 x load in kg) + (1.850 x level in cm) - (4.676 x age in years)
For men, BMR = 66.47 + (13.75 x load in kg) + (5.003 x level in cm) - (6.755 x age in years)
When you get up and start to move around, you should change this figure as you exhaust more energy.
 This worth, called Dynamic METABOLIC RATE (AMR), is determined by duplicating your BMR by an allotted number addressing the different movement levels. This number ranges from 1.2 for being inactive up to 1.9 for being extremely dynamic.
Ascertain your AMR by increasing your BMR and by your ongoing degree of action.
Stage 2: Compute Your AMR
Stationary (next to zero activity): AMR = BMR x 1.2

Daintily dynamic (practice 1-3 days/week): AMR = BMR x 1.375

Decently dynamic (practice 3-5 days/week): AMR = BMR x 1.55

Dynamic (practice 6-7 days/week): AMR = BMR x 1.725

Exceptionally dynamic (hard activity 6-7 days/week): AMR = BMR x 1.9

Your AMR addresses the quantity of calories you want to consume every day to remain at your current weight. To get thinner, you want to expand your degree of active work or decline your caloric admission by eating less.

Chapter 4

The most effective method to manage Sugar desires

For what reason do we desire Sugar?

There are many justifications for why we go for sweet things.

Starches invigorate the arrival of the vibe great mind synthetic serotonin. Sugar is starch, yet carbs(sugar molecules) come in different structures, as well, like entire grains, natural products, and vegetables, which have fiber and supplements your body needs.

The flavor of sugar likewise delivers endorphins that quiet and loosen us up.

Desserts simply taste great, as well.

Furthermore, that tendency gets built up when you reward yourself with sweet treats, which can cause you to need them significantly more. With all that making it work, is there any valid reason why we wouldn't desire sugar?

The issue comes not when we enjoy a sweet treat every so often, but when we go overboard. That is not difficult to do when sugar is added to many handled food sources, including bread, yogurt, squeezes, and sauces. Also, Americans truly do gorge it, averaging 17 teaspoons of added sugars each day, as per the American Heart Affiliation, which prescribes restricting added sugars to around 6 teaspoons each day for ladies and 9 for men.

Instructions to stop sugar desires
1. Keep your glucose levels stable:
Stable glucose levels can assist with forestalling sugar desires. To assist with keeping your glucose levels stable, don't skip dinners and ensure you incorporate low-glycemic (GI) record food in your feasts and tidbits. Food varieties with a low GI are processed and retained gradually by your body, prompting a progressive ascent in your glucose levels. This balances out your glucose levels and keeps them from spiking and dropping. Food sources with a low GI incorporate oats, wholegrain bread, quinoa, yam, lentils, beans, milk, yogurt, and many natural products including bananas, mandarins, kiwis, mangos, and pears.

2. Eat high-fiber food varieties:
Solvent fiber, which is tracked down in natural products, veggies, and grains (like oats, vegetables, and seeds), grows with water in your stomach and assists you with feeling full. It can balance out your glucose levels and assist with dealing with your sugar desires. Attempt to devour a high-fiber food with every feast. This chia pudding can be twofold as breakfast and a treat.

3. Try not to keep desserts in the house
While you don't have to stay away from your special sweet treats out and out, it tends to be more straightforward to deal with your sugar desires if you don't keep them at home. All things considered, have sound nibble choices at home prepared to eat. Assuming you have children, take a stab at getting the entire family engaged with food prep and cooking. Heat your sound biscuits or slash up some new natural products together.

4. Track down the justification behind your sugar desires
Is it true or not that you are longing for sugar since you skirted a feast and need something to eat, or is it because of stress, sleepiness, or fatigue? If it's for an explanation other than evident craving, for example, weariness, this is called eagerness for non-eating or 'brain yearning' and you want to address this first.
Assuming you are exhausted, find something non-food related that you can do to keep your brain engaged. Assuming you are worried, eliminate yourself from the distressing climate and accomplish something that can assist with diminishing your feelings of anxiety; take a walk, get some outside air, stand by listening to some music, converse with a companion, or look for assistance of a wellbeing proficient who can assist you with dealing with your pressure.

5. Eat protein-based snacks
Protein settles your glucose levels and keeps you feeling full, which can assist with decreasing your sugar desires. Incorporate a protein source in your bites like low-fat Greek yogurt or a small bunch of nuts.

6. Try not to stay away from natural product
The organic product incorporates normal sugars with different supplements like fiber, nutrients, minerals, enemies of oxidants, and phytochemicals. Because of the fiber content of the organic product, your body processes the sugar in organic products contrastingly to food varieties that are high in handled sugar. Certain individuals stress over the sugar in organic products, yet the solid measures of normal sugar it contains can thusly assist with dealing with your sugar desires.

7. Move your body
Assuming you're probably going to float towards a sweet bite straight after work, have a go at going for a stroll around then. Getting your body going delivers endorphins and helps increment your serotonin levels, causing you to feel more joyful and thus decreasing desires. Supplanting sugar with another propensity, for example, strolling will serve to decondition yourself so your mind no longer connects that season of day with sugar.
8. Hydrate

Drying out can frequently be mistaken for sugar desires. On the off chance that you feel a hankering coming on, drink a major glass of water and afterward re-evaluate assuming you are as yet needing sugar. It may very well be thirst, all things considered.
Food sources That Can Assist with forestalling Desires for Sugar:

Try not to let desires for sugar hold up traffic of your wellbeing objectives. This rundown of 20 food sources will assist with fulfilling your yearning, controlling your glucose, and assist with keeping sugar desires under control.
1. Berries
2. Avocado
3. Pistachios
4. Sesame Seeds
5. Chia Seeds
6. Quinoa
7. Oats
8. Beans and Lentils
9. Hummus
10. Coconut Oil
11. Olives and Olive Oil
12. Nonstarchy Vegetables
13. Yams
14. Greek Yogurt
15. Meat, Poultry, and Fish
16. Eggs

17. Cheddar
18. Spirulina
19. Dim Chocolate
20. Medjool Dates

Chapter 5

How to Survive Gym Shyness

What is Gym Shyness?

Gym Shyness portrays the nervousness of going to the gym or working out in a fitness center. The vast majority have this impression whenever they first step foot into a fitness office. The basic justification for this tendency is that you don't have the foggiest idea of what's in store.

Nervousness is described by sensations of strain, stressed contemplations, and actual changes, as an expanded pulse. Sensations of tension can be achieved by the unknown, similar to the primary day of school, the main day at a new position, or in any event, going to a fitness center or fitness class interestingly.

The unknown entices your creative mind to roam free and your contemplations to go into overdrive: Will it be pressed? Will everybody be more fit than me? Will individuals be great? Will they judge me for not being just about as fit as them? Will there be somebody at the front work area to converse with? What do I do if I can't track down a representative? Will they park there? Consider the possibility that I can't track down the entry. On the off chance that you've at any point had tension over another circumstance, you've probably entered this sort of thought twisting with vast inquiries that cause the pulse to keep on spiking. It tends to deplete.

One more kind of gym shyness that some experience has to do with the unknown concerning your genuine exercise. This is particularly evident when another person is composing your exercises, similar to a fitness coach or gathering health specialist.

I had these sentiments routinely as a Division I understudy competitor. As I sat in class, my stomach would do flips as I thought about the number of runs that we'd need to run during molding. What sort of mindset will the mentor be in today? Can I stroll after lifting? Or then again brush my hair? I'd feel sickened as I pondered. Right up to the present day, going to another exercise class evokes sensations of vulnerability and anxiety even though I'm capable with regards to working out.

Albeit the two situations are very normal (tension about beginning at another gym, or shyness about your booked exercise), there are steps that you can take to beat the nervousness and flourish in your fitness plan.

5 Tips for Getting Over Gym Shyness

Things being what they are, how might you beat Gym shyness? The following are five procedures that you can attempt today:

1. Know Before You Go

Since the fundamental element of Gym shyness is the unknown, you can recover control of the circumstance by getting ready before you go. This is especially useful when you're new to an office. Look at the site to find photographs, staff data (to assist you with perceiving countenances), and all broad data about the fitness center.

This can assist you with sorting out what questions you could have early so you can either call ahead and ask or record them to take with you when you visit. It tends to be useful to understand what the hours are, where to stop, whether you want an arrangement to converse with somebody, what the Coronavirus conventions are in the fitness center, and whatever else you could have to be aware of before coming in. This additional step will take out a portion of the pressure related with looking at another fitness center interestingly.

2. In-depth Relaxing

In-depth breathing can help your sensory system unwind and bring tension side effects down to nothing. One of my breathing activities is known as "box relaxing". Breathe in for 4 seconds, pause your breathing for 4 seconds, breathe out for 4 seconds (breathing out all air), and pause your breathing for 4 seconds.

When you become familiar with the example, you can build the chance to 5, 6, or even 8 seconds to assist you with unwinding. Recapitulate however long required.

3. Genuinely influence your Viewpoint

At the point when I was learning strategies for beating apprehension when it came to sports, public talking, or whatever else that can cause shyness, I discovered that viewpoint is everything. You can't help your body's reaction to the climate, yet you can channel that reaction for your benefit!

At the point when you feel those recognizable apprehensive/restless sentiments, you'll see that they feel oddly like fervor. Heart hustling, palms perspiring, expanded pulse. I bet you'd feel those equivalent sentiments hanging tight at the air terminal for a friend or family member that you haven't seen in some time! I realize I have. At the point when you feel those recognizable sentiments, rather than pondering how restless you are, tell yourself (without holding back or in your mind), "I'm so energized! This will be perfect!".

It sounds messy, however, this basic viewpoint shift is strong in assisting you with outfitting those sentiments to apply them to your advantage. You'll have a radiance in your eye when you are welcomed at the front entryway, and you can begin your exercise already having some additional increase in normal energy because of the physiological reaction to stress. Who needs caffeinated drinks, at any rate?

4. **Utilize the friend Framework**

Going to the fitness center with a friend can be very encouraging in other circumstances. It's far superior assuming that companion as of now goes to the fitness center that you're joining! They'll feel comfortable around and have an idea of the most proficient method to utilize the machines and how to explore fitness center manners.

5. **Ask Your Coach or Gathering Health specialist about the Blueprint**

While your coach or gathering educator may not give you the specific program you're doing quite a bit early, they'd probably assist you with setting your assumptions for what's to come. Your coach is probably going to have delineated an overall movement plan for you in light of your objectives and where you're beginning. They can assist you with understanding what period of preparation you're in, what kinds of activities to expect, and how lengthy you'll be in that stage so you can intellectually get ready.

In bunch wellness, you'll find that the exercises change frequently, yet the style of exercise is reliable. This can assist you with setting your assumption for impending classes even though each class could differ in trouble. In the event that you're thinking about taking a class at the fitness center, talk with the teacher to figure out what's in store as you take their class. You could try and come to the rec center when the class is happening to look into it and check whether it could work for you. In any case, you won't be aware until you attempt it.

Step-by-step instructions to Settle in working out
At the point when you're simply beginning, it's ideal to begin gradually to become accustomed to your new daily schedule. Here are a few basic hints that you can follow to get everything rolling and settle in:
1. Get a visit through the office and assist in figuring out how to utilize the machines as a whole.

2. Employ a mentor.
They'll have the option to direct you and deal with responsibilities and back you during your fitness process.

3. On the other hand, exercise with a companion. Reward if your companion knows how to put an extraordinary gym routine together.

4. Begin little and assemble your everyday practice over the long haul. Focus on a couple of days a

week and construct it over the long run. You don't need to change everything simultaneously.

5. Wear garments that you feel good in. This might appear to be irregular, yet sorting out what to wear

at the fitness center can be a tremendous wellspring of stress for some individuals. I suggest wearing agreeable garments that you can move in securely (without stressing over a piece of clothing tumbling down, tumbling off, or getting found out in a machine). Try not to stress over the most recent patterns. You're bound to be steady and sure if you're agreeable.

How regular is Fitness Center intimidation?

One more term that you might have heard before is gymtimidation. Basically, Gymtimidation is the anxiety toward working out before other people who might show up further developed or fitter than you. Gymtimidation is normal to the point that a notable rec center establishment involves it as a feature of their showcasing ploy.

The key to defeating gymtimidation is realizing that everybody in the rec center is more centered around themselves than they are on you. I don't truly intend that in a not-so-great kind of way, I essentially imply that every individual is likely there considering their objectives. Almost certainly, other fitness center participants are considering your thought process of them than deciding what you're doing.

If gymtimidation has been quite difficult for you before, it can assist with grinning and expressing hey to somebody assuming you visually engage. Generosity goes quite far in any climate, and on the off chance that you get a grin back, the terrorizing element will be brought down. Try not to be outraged on the off chance that somebody doesn't grin back, however, they may very well be in an extreme set! You can likewise chase down a generally tranquil region in the rec center to get some protection during your exercise.

Chapter 6

The Significance of Rest and Recuperation

Practice is a significant part of a sound way of life, rest and recuperation are similarly as significant. Whether you're an expert competitor or appreciate remaining dynamic, getting some margin to rest and recuperate from practice is pivotal for your general well-being and execution. We will examine the significance of rest and recuperation in training, and how you can integrate it into your daily schedule to accomplish your fitness objectives.

If you are practicing routinely and asking why you simply aren't getting in shape, in other words working on strength or not working on your performance as expected, it very well might be because you're not permitting sufficient rest and recuperation into your program.

Rest and recuperation are "a pleasant break from your program", yet a fundamental piece of your activity system that is arranged and conscious.

The reasons are 2 overlays:
Development in your muscles, first and foremost, happens when you rest, not when you work out. Working out, particularly strength preparation causes

micro tears in the muscles that your body needs to fix and adjust.

Subsequently, the transformation makes you somewhat more grounded than before so you can adapt to more load from here on out. Nonetheless, this interaction takes time, 48-72 hours, contingent upon the sort of action you do. Deficient recuperation time between practice meetings (particularly an absence of rest) doesn't permit this transformation to happen, and that implies that you don't improve or begin to injure yourself, going in reverse.

In this way, the explanation you rest is with the goal that you can prepare more and get more out of the instructional courses when you do prepare, at last, improved results.

What's more, rest permits you to renew your glycogen stores (momentary energy supply in your muscles and liver, used when you work out).

This is exhausting during exercise, particularly during cardio workouts. Sufficient nourishment and time (48 hours) permit these stores to be renewed and prepared for your next instructional meeting. Once more, the point is to work on your capacity to prepare more enthusiastically during your meetings and work on the outcomes from your preparation in the long haul.

Besides, the absence of rest and recuperation tosses your chemical levels out of equilibrium. Preparing is a "stressor", intentionally intended to stack your muscles to drive the need to adjust by delivering more development chemicals that invigorate development. In any case, your body can't distinguish between the stressors of preparing and the stressors of life, raising your regular cortisol levels.

The absence of "life stress the executives", particularly the absence of good quality rest prompts unfortunate insulin responsiveness, diminished levels of a chemical related to craving concealment (leptin), and expanded levels of a chemical related to hunger (ghrelin). This implies that you are probably going to hold muscle to fat ratio, regardless of the amount you train, and neglect to adjust to prepare true to form (The inverse of what you are attempting to accomplish).

Your objective for your preparation program ought to be to accomplish extraordinary consistency of explicit and compelling preparation by limiting life stressors and expanding your preparation load while staying in an express that considers consistent, positive transformation. The best way to accomplish this is through sufficient rest, recuperation, and great quality wholesome to help your preparation.

The following are five different ways you can integrate rest and recuperation into your work-out everyday practice:

Take Rest Days

Taking rest days is a fundamental piece of a balanced work-out everyday practice. This implies offering your body a reprieve from extreme exercises and permitting it to recuperate and fix. You can in any case remain dynamic on rest days, hold back nothing, and influence exercises like yoga, extending, or a relaxed walk.

Get Satisfactory Rest

Rest is basic for physical and mental recuperation. Hold back nothing long periods of rest every night to give your body sufficient opportunity to fix and recover. Quality rest can likewise assist with working on your concentration and state of mind, which can emphatically affect your exhibition in later exercises.

Stretch and Froth Roll

Extending and froth rolling is significant for advancing adaptability, diminishing muscle snugness, and further developing the bloodstream. This can assist with accelerating recuperation and forestall injury. Make a point to extend after every exercise and frothroll a couple of times each week to target explicit muscle gatherings.

Knead and Active recuperation

Knead and active recuperation can assist with diminishing muscle pressure and advancing the bloodstream, which can accelerate recuperation. Normal back rubs or visits to an actual specialist can likewise help distinguish and address any uneven characteristics or weak spots that might add to injury.

Pay attention to Your Body

At last, it's critical to pay attention to your body. If you feel exhausted or experience agony or distress, enjoy some time off and permit your body to rest and recuperate. Disregarding these admonition signs can prompt overtraining, injury, and diminished execution.

Conclusion

"Fleecy to Fit": All that you require to be familiar with well-being and fat misfortune," the Writer skillfully directs perusers through the intricacies of the well-being and weight of the executives. This comprehensive manual confers important information and noteworthy direction, highlighting the meaning of a balanced methodology to accomplish all-encompassing prosperity.

By focusing on the idea of complete well-being, this book prepares its perusers to go with taught choices and take on a better lifestyle, delivering it as a fundamental device for those looking to show a way towards upgraded wellness and health.